CHIROPRACTIC SPOTLIGHTS

Conversations With America's Leading Chiropractors

CHIROPRACTIC SPOTLIGHTS

Conversations With America's Leading Chiropractors

Featuring:

Dr. Jordan Burns

Dr. Andrea Esau

Dr. Mike Genslinger

Dr. Jason Pape

Dr. Keta Patel

Dr. Debra Pavlovic

Dr. Ian Rainey

Remarkable Press™

Royalties from the retail sales of **"CHIROPRACTIC SPOTLIGHTS: CONVERSATIONS WITH AMERICA'S LEADING CHIROPRACTORS"** are donated to The Global Autism Project:

AUTISM KNOWS **NO BORDERS;**
FORTUNATELY NEITHER DO WE.®

The Global Autism Project 501(C)3, is a nonprofit organization which provides training to local individuals in evidence-based practice for individuals with autism. The Global Autism Project believes that every child has the ability to learn and their potential should not be limited by geographical bounds.

The Global Autism Project seeks to eliminate the disparity in service provision seen around the world by providing high-quality training to individuals providing services in their local community. This training is made sustainable through regular training trips and contiguous remote training.

You can learn more about The Global Autism Project by visiting **GlobalAutismProject.org**

Chiropractic Spotlights/ Mark Imperial —1st ed.

Managing Editor/ Shannon Buritz

ISBN-13: 978-1-7323763-5-9

TALE OF CONTENTS

A NOTE TO THE READER

Thank you for buying your copy of "CHIROPRACTIC SPOTLIGHTS: Conversations With America's Leading Chiropractors." This book was originally created as a series of live interviews, that's why it reads like a series of conversations, rather than a traditional book that talks at you.

I wanted you to feel as though the participants and I are talking with you, much like a close friend, or relative, and felt that creating the material this way would make it easier for you to grasp the topics and put them to use quickly, rather than wading through hundreds of pages.

So relax, grab a pen and paper, take notes and get ready to immerse yourself in Chiropractic Spotlights.

Warmest regards,

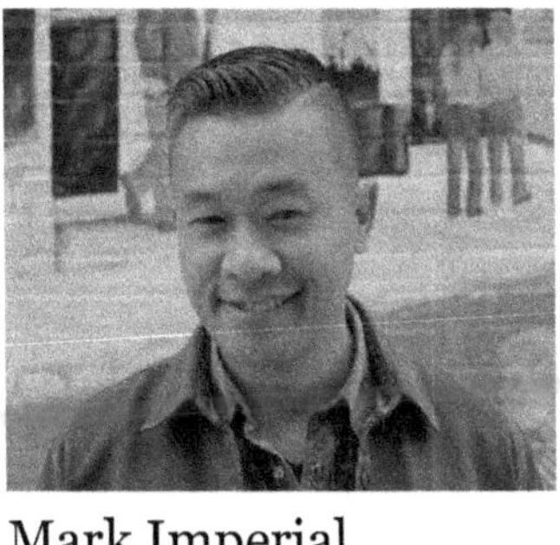

Mark Imperial
Publisher, Author and Radio Personality

INTRODUCTION

"CHIROPRACTIC SPOTLIGHTS: Conversations With America's Leading Chiropractors" is a collaborative book series featuring leading Chiropractors from across the country.

Remarkable Press™ would like to extend a heartfelt thank you to all participants who took the time to submit their chapter and offer their support in becoming ambassadors for this project.

100% of the royalties from the retail sales of this book will be donated to The Global Autism Project. Should you want to make a direct donation, visit their website at: GlobalAutismProject.org

DR. JORDAN BURNS, DC, MS

Educate the Public. Empower the Patient.

Conversation with Dr. Jordan Burns, DC, MS

Tell us about your practice and the type of patients you serve:

Dr. Jordan Burns: I help individuals become pain free with improved range of motion. I strongly believe in the value of education and provide my clients with information to make them feel more empowered in their own health care. My primary goal is to assist my clients in achieving a better quality of life. Chiropractic adds life to your years and years to your life.

What is the most common concern or challenge you hear from patients when they come to see you?

Dr. Jordan Burns*:* Most commonly, chiropractic patients come into the office feeling neglected and unheard by other providers. They have a primary complaint with no diagnosis and this often leaves them frustrated and discouraged. At this juncture, they benefit from someone shaking their hand, looking them in the eye and simply listening. The typical first time client just wants answers. They want to know the root cause of the issue, how I can help, and how long it will take to achieve improved quality of life.

What do you feel are the biggest myths out there when it comes to Chiropractic?

Dr. Jordan Burns*:* The biggest existing myths are that chiropractic care is a "quick fix" or that once you go to a chiropractor, you have to "keep going back." The term "doctor" means "to teach", so it is our duty as health care providers to educate our patients on the importance of any/all healthcare professions and the benefits associated with each.

What are some common misconceptions patients have about going through Chiropractic treatment or Chiropractic in general?

Dr. Jordan Burns*:* The most common misconception about chiropractic care is when someone states that they "threw their back out" or that "something is out of place" and the chiropractor just needs to "put it back." You aren't dislocating things in your back. Most people have the issues that they have because they are either too stagnant or too repetitive in their daily lives. They have compression or lack of mobility and chiropractic care, along with exercises/stretches, helps to combat all of these issues.

What are some of the most common fears about Chiropractic?

Dr. Jordan Burns*:* In cases of elderly patients, they often believe they are past the point of help or that they are too frail and chiropractic care might hurt. That is certainly not the case. Sure, joints degenerate over time and I'm not going to regrow discs in someone's back. However, they still have joints and can benefit from decompression and more gentle techniques to maintain the existing integrity of those joints. In general, patients often have fears about chiropractic "not working" to alleviate the issue. After fulfilling an initial care plan, if chiropractic care "doesn't work", a referral would be made for more in depth imaging/tests. I have rarely found this to be necessary.

Another common fear involves risk and/or pain associated with chiropractic care. First of all, there are no damaging side effects. The most common complaint after receiving care for the first time is initial muscle soreness, which is to be expected. As long as the proper patient consultation and examination has been performed, there are no personal risks. Even the extremely low risk of neck manipulation causing a stroke has been debunked by research.

Lastly, patients have a tendency to worry about "what others might think" of their decision to receive chiropractic care. I am a huge advocate for believing in yourself and the decisions you make regarding your personal well being. It is YOUR life. It is YOUR body. It is YOUR health.

How can they get past these fears?

Dr. Jordan Burns*:* The only way that patients can get past their fears is by our entire profession standing together to educate the masses. People don't know what they don't know. They didn't go to chiropractic school. They don't know anything about it unless we collectively make it our mission to inform them. We have to find unique ways to engage with people in order to educate them about the importance of chiropractic care.

What other perceived obstacles do you see that might be preventing people from seeking the help of a Chiropractor?

Dr. Jordan Burns*:* People are often under the false impression that chiropractic care will "cost too much". On the contrary, chiropractic care is typically less expensive than a "normal" doctor's visit. Considering the costs of potential pharmaceutical drugs and surgeries associated with traditional alternatives, a chiropractic care plan ends up being far less expensive.

In addition, we live in a society that thrives on "instant gratification". People need to understand that chiropractic care isn't a "quick fix". As stated previously, most people have issues due to long-standing habits of being too stagnant or too repetitive in their daily lives. It takes time for decompression, chiropractic adjustments and corrective exercises to have long-term and long-lasting effects on the human body.

What are some of the little known pitfalls or common mistakes you see people make when seeking Chiropractic treatment? How can these be avoided?

Dr. Jordan Burns*:* The biggest pitfall is patients having unrealistic expectations when it comes to receiving care. When common phrases like "I threw my back out" are used during the first visit, it gives the notion that something is "out" and I need to put it back. In the patient's mind, this should be a quick, easy, one time fix. This is simply not the case. In order to avoid expectations like this, patient education is as crucial as ever in order for the chiropractic profession to thrive as it is intended to. There must be an emphasis on relationship building with each patient on the first and second visits to establish trust and clear communication about the diagnosis and treatment plan.

Can you share an example of how you have helped a patient overcome these obstacles and succeed in their Chiropractic treatments?

Dr. Jordan Burns*:* My first two visits with patients consist of educating them on their primary complaint, their diagnosis, their treatment plan and how chiropractic care can help. I had a 47 year old male patient come in recently who had never been to a chiropractor before. He talked about how he "threw his back out." I ask every patient what their goals are upon stepping into my office. His goal for treatment was for me to "put him back together." Although I can obviously empathize and understand where he is coming from with this vernacular, I also immediately began to educate him on the fact that nothing was displaced or dislocated in his back. Once again, this sets us on the path to realistic expectations when it comes to treatment. An informed patient is better able to recognize and embrace the benefits of care.

What inspired you to become a Chiropractor?

Dr. Jordan Burns: It started back when I was a sprinter in college and I had a rib subluxation during a weightlifting session. I had the worst debilitating mid back pain after this and I couldn't take a deep breath without pain. I had soft tissue work done in our training room but it didn't seem like it was enough. I researched and decided to seek out chiropractic care for the first time. After one adjustment, I stood up and was completely pain free. I thought to myself, "What is this witchcraft?" After a few more visits, I asked if I could shadow that doctor and I inevitably changed career paths because of it. Chiropractic was the hidden profession for me. Even as a kid, I understood the general concept of chiropractic. I understood that when I was sick, my body wasn't deficient in any drug. I wasn't sleeping enough, drinking enough fluids, taking the proper vitamins and minerals etc. My body was designed to heal from the inside out.

Every day, I feel like my body is going to explode with love, energy and compassion for people. It is my mission to preach and teach chiropractic care, love, positivity, personal development, humility, and kindness until I no longer have the ability to do so. I make it a point to work on myself every day and share that journey with people to the best of my ability. To serve others. To teach others. To empower others.

Can you share a lesson you learned early on, that still impacts how you do business today?

Dr. Jordan Burns*:* The only way to truly believe and understand the power of the chiropractic profession is to see it firsthand. For me, it was hard early on to suggest long-term care plans to people until I could fully understand how absolutely necessary chiropractic care is for the function of the human body. It comes with time. It comes with practice. It comes with patience.

What's the most important question people should ask themselves as they consider Chiropractic?

Dr. Jordan Burns*:* What are you goals for your life and your overall health? Do you want to simply live or do you want to THRIVE?

What's the most important thing people should consider when evaluating a Chiropractor?

Dr. Jordan Burns*:* What are your goals for care and do the chiropractor's treatment methods line-up with those goals? Evaluate their website, Google reviews and call their office if you have any questions before scheduling an appointment.

How can someone find out more about you, your practice, how you can help, and how to reach you?

Dr. Jordan Burns*:* The best ways to contact/communicate with me are via social media, specifically Instagram, @DrJordanBurns or email me at jordanburnsdc@gmail.com. I am always more than willing to help in any way that I can Thank you from the bottom of my heart for reading.

DR. JORDAN BURNS, DC, MS

Owner/Chiropractor

ProWellness Chiropractic

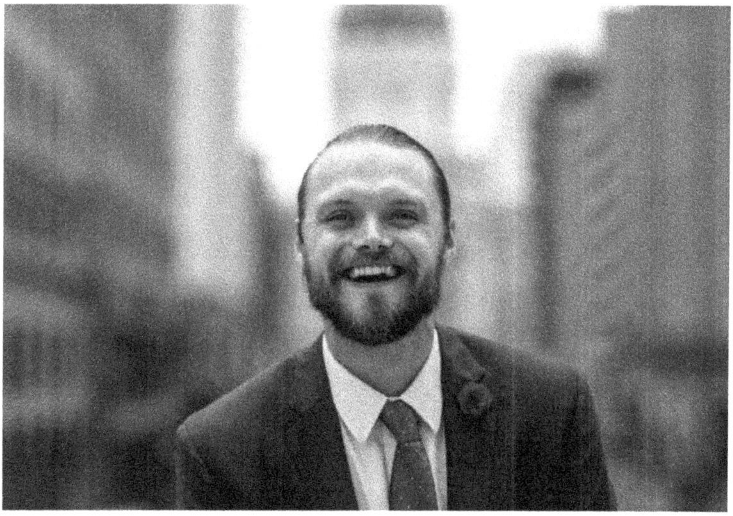

Dr. Jordan Burns is a practicing chiropractor in the greater Indianapolis, Indiana area. He was born and raised in southern Indiana. He grew up in Oakland City, where he enjoyed many years of basketball, football, soccer, and track and field. Being involved in so many extracurricular sports is where he first realized how his love for sports performance and fitness could lead to a career.

Fulfilling a childhood dream, Dr. Burns attended Indiana University-Bloomington where he received his first Bachelor's degree in Kinesiology. While being a member of the men's track and field team at Indiana, he suffered from back pain after a weight-lifting incident. After going to a local chiropractor for the first time ever, he was finally pain free after his adjustment. He decided to switch career paths after researching and experiencing the benefits of chiropractic care firsthand.

Dr. Burns then moved to St. Louis, Missouri where he attended Logan University-College of Chiropractic, graduating with a Bachelor's in Life Sciences, a Master's in Sports Science and Rehabilitation, and his Doctorate of Chiropractic. While at Logan, Dr. Burns was accepted as a Senior Intern in the Biofreeze Human Performance Center, a clinic that specializes in sport specific injuries and rehabilitation.

Dr. Burns is board-certified by the National and Indiana Boards of Chiropractic and has enjoyed successfully treating patients in pain. He uses a variety of specific chiropractic and therapy treatment protocols that allow him and his qualified staff to provide a gentle, effective approach to many different muscular, neurological, and joint-related conditions for people of all ages.

In his personal life, Dr. Burns makes a valiant effort to practice what he preaches. He enjoys staying active by weight-lifting, running, and playing basketball. He also loves cooking and he cherishes spending time with his girlfriend, family and friends.

WEBSITE: www.DrJordanBurns.com
EMAIL: jordanburnsdc@gmail.com
LINKEDIN: www.linkedin.com/in/drjordanburns
FACEBOOK: www.facebook.com/DrJordanBurns/
TWITTER: @DrJordanBurns
INSTAGRAM: @DrJordanBurns
TIKTOK: @DrJordanBurns

DR. ANDREA ESAU

Conversation with Dr. Andrea Esau

Tell us about your practice and the type of patients you serve.

Dr. Andrea Esau*:* My practice name is Gentle Hands Healing Centre out of Roswell, Georgia. I specialize in working with children, specifically highly sensitive children. I find that many parents are wanting the benefits of chiropractic care for their kids, but in a more gentle, less startling way. About 40% of my patients are children under the age of twelve. I also see a sprinkling of people from every walk of life including teenagers, adults, seniors, and athletes.

What are the benefits of chiropractic care for children?

Dr. Andrea Esau*:* Many children these days are struggling with anxiety and depression. They may have difficulty concentrating at school or at home. It can become a struggle for them to sleep at night because of extreme anxiety and a feeling of being overwhelmed. A lot of parents come into my office and are concerned for their children because they simply do not seem happy. It is starting to have a negative impact on all aspects of daily life for the child and parents come to me in search of a solution. Chiropractic care is not just about treating pain. I can help children overcome these issues and get back to enjoying life again.

The purpose of chiropractic is to increase function of the nervous system and proprioception through the joints. Research has shown that chiropractic care can help with a number of common childhood issues including colic, anxiety and depression, asthma, attention and concentration, immune system function, sleep disturbances, and even bedwetting. When it comes to the issue of pain, especially with the rise in how much young children use technology, kids are experiencing pain in ways that we didn't see in the past. In any case, chiropractic care can have life changing results for adults and children alike.

What do you feel are the biggest myths and misconceptions out there when it comes to Chiropractic?

Dr. Andrea Esau*:* A common misconception is the amount of education it takes to become a chiropractor. Many people believe that the education, time, and intensity put in is equivalent to a one or two year program. In reality, it took me eight years to become a chiropractor. It is a rigorous, in depth program similar to what a traditional doctor would go through. We study much of the same material when it comes to anatomy and physiology, with more emphasis on chiropractic technique.

Secondly, there is a misconception when it comes to adjusting children that many parents are fearful about. They think of chiropractic as the classic, forceful neck movement or the "snap, crackle, pop", so to speak. And they become very scared about doing that to their baby or child. No chiropractic school in the country teaches to adjust children in this manner. I have an entirely different, very gentle approach for babies, small children, or even adults who desire a less forceful adjustment.

What inspired you to become a Chiropractor?

Dr. Andrea Esau*:* I was one of those kids whose life was turned completely upside down in the best possible way through getting adjusted. Right around the age of thirteen, I started having severe, debilitating back pain. It is interesting since it sounds like the beginning of a very classic chiropractic story. By the age of seventeen, the pain was getting progressively worse. I would cry every morning before school because I was just so miserable. I then started having serious migraines and heart arrhythmias. My mom brought me to every doctor and every specialist in search of answers with no luck. My parents knew this wasn't normal for a young teenage girl to be in so much pain. I had basically given up hope. Fortunately for me, my parents had not. My mom found a chiropractor over an hour away from where we lived. She took me there 3 days a week early in the morning before school started, with my little sister in tow. It was certainly a commitment...a commitment that was well worth it. I remember the feeling of sitting in the office after my adjustment as though a boulder had just been lifted from my shoulders. For the first time in years, I felt like I could breathe...like I was okay. Later that day, when I came home from school, my family was in the kitchen and my mom said something funny. I started laughing at her and my mom and sister both started crying. I didn't understand what was going on. My mom said "This is the first time we have seen you smile or laugh in years."

It was then that I knew what I wanted to do with my life. I owe my childhood chiropractor for really encouraging me to go to chiropractic school. My grades had suffered in high school since I was in so much pain all the time, and I lost confidence that I was smart enough to go to chiropractic school. She supported me and assured me I could do it and so my journey began.

Going to school and running a business is hard. You can never lose focus of why you are doing it. On the really tough days, you need something to hold onto that keeps you going. For me, it is reflecting on my high school days and thinking that if I can just help one person as much as I was helped, it will all be worth it. It truly is a great honor to be able to help so many people regain quality of life through chiropractic care.

How can someone find out more about you, your practice, how you can help, and how to reach you?

Dr. Andrea Esau: You can find out more about me on my website at www.gentlehandshealing.com. In addition, I can be found on Facebook and Instagram at Gentle Hands Healing .

DR. ANDREA ESAU, DC

Owner/Founder

Gentle Hands Healing Centre

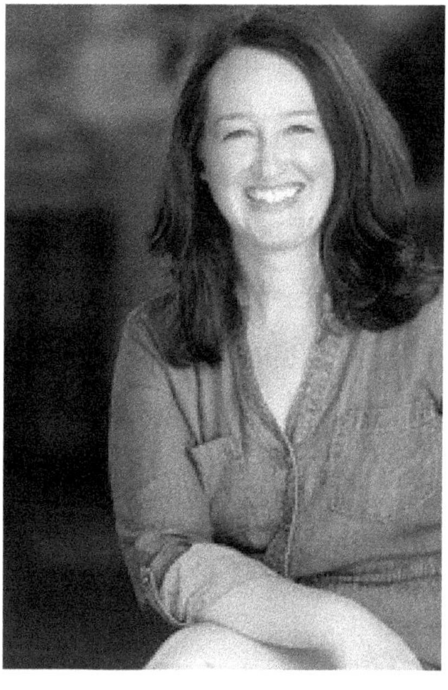

I came to love Chiropractic by experiencing the powerful healing effect it has. As a teenager I had debilitating pain and wasn't sure I'd be able to find anything that could help me. I am profoundly grateful that I did; I found Chiropractic and my life radically changed for the better.

As I continued on my journey, I discovered that Chiropractic is about so much more than recovering from pain or returning to normal. It's also about becoming healthier and stronger than you were before or maybe even more so than you ever thought possible. Chiropractic benefits people of all ages. While I love working with people of all ages and stages of life, I especially love helping moms and their children discover health!

By learning to connect with my mind and body, I discovered that I was a powerful healer and advocate for myself and that my body could learn to grow and adapt in ways that kept me feeling better overall as well as recovering faster when life threw some curveballs.

Working with moms and kids has given me an especially rewarding outlet to use my own sensitive and gentle nature to serve this community more fully!

I graduated from Life University in Marietta, Georgia in 2014 as a Doctor of Chiropractic. I also have a Bachelor's in Science in Biology from Life University. It is my greatest honor to serve this community and I would love the chance to take care of you & your family. I hope that Chiropractic becomes a part of your journey!

WEBSITE: www.gentlehandshealing.com

FACEBOOK: Gentle Hands Healing
INSTAGRAM: @gentlehandshealing

DR. MIKE GENSLINGER

Healing Naturally with DuPage Family Chiropractic

Conversation with Dr. Mike Genslinger

Tell us about your practice and the type of patients you serve.

Dr. Mike Genslinger*:* At DuPage Family Chiropractic, we are dedicated to providing our community with a solution to their health needs without the use of drugs or surgery. On a daily basis, we treat everything from neck and back pain in adults to colic and constipation in infants. The most common conditions we help with are headaches and migraines. One of the greatest contributing factors has been our increased utilization of technology. Whether it is at home or in the workplace, Americans spend at least 8 hours a day on tech devices. How does this contribute to migraines and poor health? Eye strain and increase in sedentary lifestyle often occur, but one of the greatest impacts is poor posture. We are often hunching over these devices, ultimately causing a loss of normal cervical curvature.

Short, N., Mays, M., Cool, A., Delay, A., Lannom, A., O'Donnell, L., & Stuber, R. (2020). Defining Mobile Tech Posture: Prevalence and Position Among Millennials. The Open Journal of Occupational Therapy, 8(1), 1-10. https://doi.org/10.15453/2168-6408.1640

With specific treatment plans created for each patient, we are able to achieve tremendous results. Before starting care, many patients have altered their daily living in order to “get by” with their current symptoms or condition. When starting care, many patients may be suffering from daily headaches and we bring most to a place where they are no longer experiencing them at all! Now they are able to enjoy life again, spending time with family/friends and participating in activities they enjoy. That can be as simple as going for a walk as they are no longer worried about sensitivity to the light, or enjoying a child's sporting event without concern of a cheering crowd triggering a headache/migraine. Our patients feel like they have regained their quality of life.

Patients are able to make dramatic changes to their lives after starting care. We have countless patients who have completely turned their lives around. Here is just one example:

"After experiencing severe neck and back pain for years, being told my only real option to fix it was cortisone shots and ultimately surgery, Dr. Mike was able to create a treatment and maintenance plan for me that has not only virtually eliminated the pain, but also got me off the meds that I was prescribed for it. I can't thank him enough, as the quality of my day to day life is so much better because of the work he did. Now my whole family goes to him! Thanks Dr. Mike! See you at my next visit!"

What is the most common concern or challenge you hear from patients when they come to see you?

Dr. Mike Genslinger*:* One of the most common challenges that we encounter in our office is patients who have lost hope regarding their condition. They have been to many other doctors/offices with little to no results. For some, it was their neighbor who referred them or they saw a video that chiropractic can help. They have exhausted all other options and are willing to try anything to get relief. Chiropractic is not an overnight fix and we do a very thorough job explaining the process to achieve the desired results. I wish that I was able to fix everyone with just one treatment but that is simply not the case. Many times these issues have been present for years and it will take some time to correct. We always strive to achieve quick results and something I can guarantee is that we will do everything we can to get patients performing their best as fast as possible.

What do you feel are the biggest myths out there when it comes to Chiropractic?

Dr. Mike Genslinger: A common skepticism we hear in the field of chiropractic care is "Are you even a real doctor?" To be clear, doctors of chiropractic receive more training in anatomy and physiology, while physicians or MDs receive more training in areas like obstetrics and psychology. Chiropractic colleges focus on chiropractic principles, diagnosis, orthopedics, physiologic therapeutics and nutrition. There are certain areas such as manipulative/adjustive techniques, spinal analysis, physical/clinical laboratory diagnosis and diagnosis imaging that account for more than half of the education. During their internship, doctors of chiropractic complete two years of hands-on clinical experience focusing on manipulation/adjustment as the primary treatment procedure. This can be done either in the student clinic located on campus or through formal training under the supervision of a practicing chiropractor in a private clinic setting. Comparison studies show that chiropractic education actually devotes more time to the basic and clinical sciences than do medical schools. So yes, we are real doctors.

https://biology.uni.edu/sites/default/files/chiropractic_education_vs_medical_education.pdf

What are some common misconceptions patients have about going through Chiropractic treatment or Chiropractic in general?

Dr. Mike Genslinger*:* One of the biggest misconceptions is that the adjustment is going to hurt. With specific manipulation of a joint properly performed by a trained chiropractor, the adjustment will not hurt. I will say, as with any manual therapy work, side effects may be present after the manipulation. Soreness or tenderness may occur but will resolve within 24-48 hours. I always tell my patients that it is very similar to starting a new workout program. You may be sore for a day or so after your first adjustment, but once we get the joints moving better, that will not happen anymore. I have found this to be a good analogy that everyone can understand because at one point in our lives we have all experienced this.

What are some of the most common fears about Chiropractic?

Dr. Mike Genslinger*:* One of the most common fears revolves around one of the most common misconceptions...that the adjustment is going to cause pain. This is not the case at all! There are many different techniques when it comes to adjusting and I use a technique called Prone Specific. This is a very light and gentle approach that does not use a lot of pressure. I only need to move the joints 1-2mm in order to gain the desired results. Our patients love this technique because they can be very relaxed for their adjustment and not have to worry about the excess pressure or force that some techniques require. In fact, we feel that we achieve better results using this specific technique.

How can patients get past these fears?

Dr. Mike Genslinger*:* Ultimately, they have to give it a try in order to see for themselves how safe chiropractic adjustments are. Also, the results speak for themselves as demonstrated by the following data. In a comparative-effectiveness trial, 94% of manual-thrust manipulation (chiropractic) recipients experienced a reduction in their pain, compared with only 54% of medical care recipients (prescription medication). Chiropractors are the highest-rated healthcare practitioner for low-back pain treatments above physical therapists (PTs), specialist physician/MD (i.e., neurosurgeons, neurologists, orthopaedic surgeons), and primary care physician/MD (i.e., family or internal medicine).

https://www.acatoday.org/News-Publications/Newsroom/Key-Facts

What other perceived obstacles do you see that might be preventing people from seeking the help of a Chiropractor?

Dr. Mike Genslinger*:* An obstacle that we must strive to overcome with many patients is the cost of care. We try our best to make it affordable for everyone with a variety of payment options. We will even offer free financing in house for up to 12 months. Once patients start to experience and feel the difference chiropractic can make in their lives, most do not want to stop. We see many patients participating in activities they only dreamed about without any limitations.

Secondly, time limitations that patients have for treatment is often an obstacle. In order to be respectful of our patients' busy schedules, we are very efficient and take a different approach than many other offices. Physical therapy is a necessary component to our treatment plans, but our patients perform this primarily in the comfort of their own homes, on their schedule instead of in the office. When a patient starts care we are now in agreement that I will do everything I can for them in the office and they need to do their part by performing exercises at home. Not only is this time efficient for them, but it also increases accountability for their own health. The office visit time is dramatically decreased and they have the flexibility to fit the exercises in anytime they wish. Patients love this plan as many come on their lunch break and are able to get back to work within a reasonable timeframe. Encouraging healthy habits at home is a very important component of our practice and the care we provide.

What are some of the little known pitfalls or common mistakes you see people make when seeking Chiropractic treatment? How can these be avoided?

Dr. Mike Genslinger*:* Oftentimes patients will try to determine for themselves whether or not they need more treatment based solely on how they feel. There is a difference between feeling good and staying stable. Patients are so excited to move better and feel better that they jump right back into normal activities. This is where we run into problems. Pain is not a good way to judge if you need additional treatment or not. Pain is one of the last symptoms to present itself. Essentially, it is one of the last things to show up but the first to leave. I always have to remind my patients to take it easy and allow for the joints to stabilize before getting back to normal activities. We don't ever want to start from scratch and diminish progress simply because a patient does too much over the weekend.

This can be avoided by talking with your doctor and creating a maintenance plan. Exercise is a very simple concept I use to help patients understand the importance of maintenance. For example, when you reach your fitness goal, can you stop exercising completely and maintain everything you worked so hard for? No...and the exact same goes for chiropractic. The majority of our patients who start maintenance plans will come either every other week or one time per month.

Can you share an example of how you have helped a patient overcome these obstacles and succeed in their Chiropractic treatments?

Dr. Mike Genslinger*:* Here is a testimonial from one of our maintenance patients who now understands the principles of chiropractic.

“I met Dr. Mike a couple of years ago and I thought...young guy, new thought process on adjustments, got the most recent technological schooling, let's give him a try. I have been PAIN FREE since starting treatment. I am glad to see a more modern approach to adjustments, meaning I don't get bent like a pretzel and smashed around. The bottom line is being FREE from chronic pain I had that has disappeared by following his treatment plan.”

This patient currently comes in once a month for his maintenance adjustment and continues to do great!

What inspired you to become a Chiropractor?

Dr. Mike Genslinger*:* I was an athlete all my life and chiropractic played a very large role in my success of staying on the field and being healthy. I always loved the feeling of walking out of the office after getting adjusted and thinking to myself "How can an adjustment do that?" I wanted to provide that same feeling for others and I made the decision to become a chiropractor back in high school. Chiropractic is so wonderful and the best part about it is that we are empowering individuals to heal naturally. We do not need any special machinery or reliance on medications. Everything that I do is simply with my two hands. One of the most rewarding parts of my profession is seeing the changes we can make in someone's life in a relatively short period of time. From having to be helped by their spouse into the office because they were having trouble walking to going on family bike rides within a few short weeks. It doesn't get much better than that!

Can you share a lesson you learned early on that still impacts how you do business today?

Dr. Mike Genslinger*:* One lesson I learned early on is that I was not connecting with my patients on the level that they deserved. What I mean by this is that I wanted everyone to like me and be my friend. I strive now to be a doctor FIRST, and then a friend. I feel honored that my patients take time out of their day to see me and put trust in me that I will do the best I can for them each visit. I try to limit conversation outside of their issue because I want them to know that when they are in my office, they have 100% of my focus on why they are here and not on the weather or who won the game last night.

What's the most important question people should ask themselves as they consider Chiropractic?

Dr. Mike Genslinger*:* They need to ask themselves if they are ready to make the change. As I have stated before, chiropractic is not an overnight fix and one visit will not fix many years of damage. If the patient can commit to making a change to improve their health,, then they are ready to start care. When patients start care and then stop after a few visits because "it didn't work for them", it is a telltale sign they were not ready to begin in the first place. When treatment protocols are followed, chiropractic has the highest satisfaction rating in terms of results with 93% according to a 2015 RAND study.

What's the most important thing people should consider when evaluating a Chiropractor?

Dr. Mike Genslinger*:* Patients should seek out a chiropractor with a philosophy that matches their own. With chiropractic, there are many different ways to practice and not all chiropractors are the same. Some may be more rehab based and perform a lot of physical therapy, while others can focus strictly on adjustments. It is important that you align yourself with someone that you feel comfortable with and can put your trust in.

How can someone find out more about you, your practice, how you can help, and how to reach you?

Dr. Mike Genslinger*:* We can always be found on our website at drmikegenslinger.com or by phone at 630-442-7175. We are available to answer any questions you have about your condition and how we can help!

DR. MIKE GENSLINGER

Chiropractor

Dupage Family Chiropractic

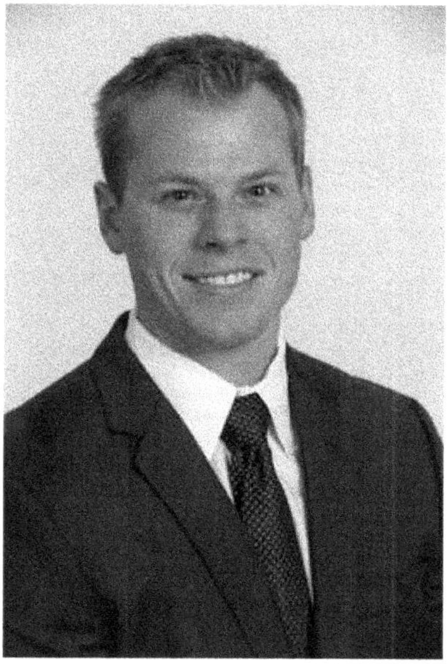

I am dedicated to enhancing daily living and improving the general well being of the Lisle community and surrounding DuPage County through exceptional chiropractic care and education. I believe in treating the body as a whole, focusing equal importance on all areas that support and build a healthy lifestyle. Patient education is a key element of this process. Providing patients with the proper educational tools to better understand their health and motivating them to take an active role in their own wellness promotes healthy living long-term. I pride myself on patient focus and satisfaction. I pledge myself to your needs in the most expedient, professional and courteous manner possible. I commit myself to listen to you so that I may understand your needs and provide you with the highest quality attention and care available. I am dedicated to your care and well-being.

Dr. Michael Genslinger was born and raised in the Chicagoland area. He is a graduate of the University of Wisconsin-Platteville and National University of Health Sciences. Dr. Genslinger has a life-long passion for athletics and played football while attending UW-Platteville. He enjoys working with patients of all age groups and holds certifications in Webster Technique, Mckenzie Parts A and B and RockTape Fascial Movement Taping Levels 1 and 2.

WEBSITE: drmikegenslinger.com

EMAIL: office@drmikegenslinger.com

LINKEDIN: linkedin.com/in/dr-mike-genslinger-a8a9b2b0

FACEBOOK: https://www.facebook.com/DuPage-Family-Chiropractic-1608354426052305

OFFICE: 630-442-7175

FAX: 630-631-0998

Conversation with Dr. Jason Pape

Tell us about your practice and the type of patients you serve.

Dr. Jason Pape: When it comes to the chiropractic side of my practice, I treat anything musculoskeletal which includes not just the spine, back, and neck, but the head, ankles, wrists, knees, and shoulders as well. I talk to my patients about viewing me as their holistic primary since I can advocate and guide them on pretty much any issue they may be struggling with. Obviously, if you are having a heart attack or break your arm in half, I won't be your first stop. But I like to be a resource to my patients regardless of the stops in their journey, providing them with answers they may not be receiving from other medical professionals.

I have a full scale practice treating patients of any age. I focus a lot of my time and energy on pediatrics, from newborns on up. Parents often are in search of help for issues like colic, reflux, GERD, ear infections, and other chronic conditions. I can help with many of these issues when parents are seeking an alternative to medication. I also see many children with disabilities including Autism and ADHD. Chiropractic plays a large role in the well-being of babies and young children.

In addition, I have a wellness center to cover many more bases when it comes to holistic medicine. My team of other practitioners provides services like acupuncture, massage therapy, hypnotherapy, psychotherapy, yoga, Reiki, nutrition, and more. All of these alternative options often help our patients gain relief without having to resort to drugs or surgery.

I pride myself on understanding functional medicine and the ability to heal the body with nutrition, diet, and lifestyle. When something is wrong with our body or we are experiencing a chronic illness, we don't necessarily need to cut something out, inject it, or load it up with pills. We simply need to find the root of the problem and rectify it naturally. All of the systems in our body work together intimately as one unit. Sometimes, traditional medical professionals become so specialized that they only focus on one area. By focusing on the entire body and the communication between each system, we can help patients reach their optimal level of health and utilize methods to help the body heal itself.

What is the most common concern or challenge you hear from pediatric patients?

Dr. Jason Pape*:* When it comes to my pediatric patients, I see many babies who are colicky. These are infants who simply will not stop crying and are irritated all the time. As you can imagine, these parents are on the verge of ripping their hair out trying to find a way to help their child. In a similar vein are the babies who are spitting up a lot. They have chronic reflux or ear infections and are being medicated for these issues. In our office we have found that chiropractic care seems to be extremely helpful with many conditions. Often, things happen to create these issues starting all the way from birth. Was the baby delivered vaginally? If so, was it an easy delivery or were forceps involved? Instruments like forceps are very impactful on the neck and spine, especially on a tiny baby weighing only eight or nine pounds. On the contrary, we have the babies who were delivered via C-section. They don't get the advantage of coming through the birth canal and the spinal and cranial molding that comes along with that. Not to mention, they are pulled out of the womb by their head. All of these things could cause the spine to be subluxated and not moving properly. The only way a baby can communicate any issues is to cry.

I perform a very gentle type of adjusting on small babies. I do not twist or crack little baby spines. I manipulate them in a way that is gentle, effective, and allows the body to communicate with the brain without interference. Adjusting the spine helps torticollis, and we have seen many patients have relief from colic and even ear infections as the adjustment can open up the ear canals to allow them to drain better. From a functional medicine perspective, I also find myself talking to parents about what the mom is eating if she is breastfeeding, what type of formula or food the baby is being given, or what probiotics we could incorporate to promote gut health. All of these aspects can play a role in chronic ear infections. Once again, it is so important to be able to give my patients the WHOLE picture and get to the root cause of the particular condition.

What is the most common concern or challenge you hear from patients with special needs?

Dr. Jason Pape: Some of the most common concerns for my special needs patients are attention/focus and sensory integration issues. Most of them are receiving speech, occupational, and physical therapy, but sometimes they need more. One of the things I find is that their brains need to be integrated better. Chiropractic helps take stress off the nervous system. With conditions like ADHD, Autism, and Aspergers, children are experiencing sensory integration dysregulation. This happens when their brains are unable to properly prioritize and filter information from one or more of their eight sensory systems. An example of this would be a child trying to pay attention to the teacher in class. But the tag on the back of his shirt is itching, the kid next to him is tapping his pencil, and there is a butterfly outside the window. It becomes difficult for the child to filter and prioritize all of this input. What should he be paying attention to when the brain is telling him everything is important? We have certain exercises and modalities that we can use in the office to teach the brain to focus better to more properly integrate this aberrant sensory input. We can actually drive neuroplastic change by establishing new pathways and better connections in the brain through repetitive challenge.

This, along with dietary changes and chiropractic care, can produce amazing results for our special needs children.

With any of the pediatric patients that we see, we consider the certain primitive reflexes that we are born with. These reflexes are supposed to integrate into the system within the first twelve to twenty-four months of life in a specific order. If they don't integrate properly or are not replaced with certain postural reflexes, causing the primitive ones to remain, it can negatively affect integration and function. For example, a very basic one is called the Moro or "startle" reflex. It should integrate in the first two to four months of life. If it doesn't, it keeps you stuck in "fight or flight" mode, which causes a great deal of stress to the system. All sensory input enters at high priority because you don't know where danger is coming from. In our office, we can discover the reflexes that never integrated and force them to integrate at any age using specific exercises and maneuvers. This is beneficial to a wide variety of children, with or without special needs or diagnoses.

What is the most common concern or challenge you hear from patients with musculoskeletal issues?

Dr. Jason Pape: Low back pain, neck pain, and headaches tend to be the most common problems patients are experiencing when they walk in my door. Often, patients don't realize that chiropractic treats beyond the spine. I will hear "Well, I have ankle pain too. But I know you can't help with that." Yes, I CAN help with that!.

Recently, I had a brand new patient with a neck issue and a mid back rib issue. He had pain in his mid thoracic that was wrapping around to the front for five or six years on and off. After seeing tons of doctors and undergoing several tests, he still had no answers. One doctor did mention that it could be coming from his back, but did not provide any recourse. Within a couple minutes of him describing the pain, I knew exactly what was wrong because we see this type of situation all the time. He had rib subluxation, causing his pain to travel around his torso from back to front. Often, things that are unable to be identified or treated by traditional medicine are, in fact, very easily taken care of through chiropractic!

I often explain to my new patients who have never seen a chiropractor before that the brain and body communicate through the spinal cord. The spinal cord is housed in the spine, which is a series of bones that sit on top of each other, each having a range of motion. Nerves branch out from every segment and go to your muscles, joints, immune system, and organs. This creates a constant flow of information going back and forth from the spinal cord to the brain. If things are not moving correctly in the spine, it can cause interference in the way the nerves communicate information and lead to dysfunction. This can come in the form of muscle spasms, pain or even result in other issues. My job as a chiropractor is to find that area of spinal interference, also known as a subluxation. Upon finding it, I apply a chiropractic adjustment, which is just a small, localized force into the spine that restores normal motion. When that happens, the body can begin to heal itself. We have an innate intelligence in every cell of our body that knows what to do when it comes to healing. For example, if you cut your hand, you don't have to think about it or focus on it to get it to heal. Your body knows how to take care of it. So the goal for all of my patients is to get them to a place where the body and brain can communicate without interference, expediting healing and helping them achieve true wellness.

And remember, every joint in the body has a range of motion and can become subluxated, not just the spine! This is why we can help with many different issues beyond just the spine as we are trained to also address these areas and have the training and education to do so as well.

Also, preventative care is an important component of chiropractic. There is more to it than just resolving the pain. I always tell my patients "the absence of pain is not the presence of health." Maintenance care will help prevent little things from becoming big things. Patients who have a care plan and stick to it have less problems and bounce back faster because their body becomes used to these more proper spinal movements. In addition, their brains and bodies are communicating without dysfunctional interference. I want my patients to function at an optimal level of health long after the pain is gone.

Tell us about the use of functional medicine in your practice.

Dr. Jason Pape: I see many patients with chronic health issues such as autoimmune dysfunctions, fibromyalgia, Crohn's disease and IBS. These chronic illnesses are where something has gone wrong in the system. I have to take a look at the body and figure out why these things are happening. Our goal chiropractically is to take a load off the system. For example, let's take a look at thyroid issues. First, we will consider the patient's health history and take an in-depth look at bloodwork. We typically look at bloodwork much differently than a traditional medicine doctor would, running much more extensive thyroid blood panels. With this information, other blood work parameters, combined with a detailed patient history, we can determine how the thyroid is truly functioning and whether or not the thyroid is the main problem or a secondary issue. Often, another system could be causing the thyroid to function abnormally. In many cases, thyroid issues are secondary to other underlying problems. Patients come to me that have been diagnosed with autoimmune thyroid and their only recourse was to be given medication. They don't want to be medicated and are looking for other solutions. As we look at the other systems and how they are playing into it, we can use things like diet and nutrition to make shifts within the body. The body now starts to heal itself because we are giving it what it needs.

With most of my functional medicine patients, one of the first things I focus on is the gut. 80% of your immune system is housed in your gut. When problems arise in the gut, they can leak into other parts of the system causing inflammation, infection, and irritation. Because we have been exposed to so many things throughout our lifetimes such as unhealthy foods, antibiotics, and vaccines that kill off good bacteria, sometimes there is a lot of work to do to pull back the layers and restore the balance. As long as the patient is willing to take some of their health into their own hands, we can help. Through functional medicine, we understand our patients in a way that many traditional doctors don't. We can break the cycle of being bounced from doctor to doctor or medication to medication by finding and restoring the balance lost within the system.

What do you feel are the biggest myths out there when it comes to Chiropractic?

Dr. Jason Pape*:* Over the years, one of the most common myths I've heard is that chiropractic care is a "scam" because you "have to keep going back". When you go to a chiropractor, it's not going to be a one time thing. Nobody goes to a physical therapist expecting a one time visit. You go for four to six weeks, three times a week, until your body is healed. Injuries take time to heal. The same goes for chiropractic care. In order for me to get your body back to optimal functioning, it is going to take some repetition of care. We take care of our cars by performing routine maintenance such as oil changes. We take care of our teeth by brushing them and going to the dentist for cleanings. You don't hear people complaining about having to "keep going back" to the dentist or saying it is a "scam". You don't want to wait until you have a problem like a cavity to go to the dentist. This is the same reason why preventative chiropractic care is so important. The spine is just as important as our teeth. It houses the nervous system and you are moving, turning, and twisting every single day. You are engaging in repetitive motions and moving in ways that are improper or not ergonomically correct. It is these daily actions we return to after treatment that are part of why repetition is needed to help gain resolution, especially if someone has had a chronic issue for many years. If something has been there for many years, it doesn't usually go away overnight. The body likes what it knows, good or bad, and repetition drives change in the body. To truly resolve an issue and maintain health, a number of visits initially may be necessary followed by preventative care visits. Preventative care helps to eliminate any future problems, shorten treatment times if problems do arrive, and overall maintain a healthy spine and nervous system.

Another common misconception is that chiropractors are not "real doctors." In fact, our education is very similar to medical school. We actually receive one hundred more hours of gross anatomy than medical doctors do. Where they get pharmacology, we get more chiropractic philosophy and adjusting instruction.

Chiropractors have been put in a box for a long time. The AMA actually tried to discredit the field and shut us down in the '80s and we won a lawsuit after that attempt. Since then, chiropractic care has become much more widely accepted. When it comes to the discrepancies between traditional medicine and the functional medicine piece of what I do, I describe it as this: Traditional doctors come out of medical school with a very nice toolbox full of hammers. They are all beautiful hammers, but hammers just the same. When all you have are hammers, everything starts to look like a nail. Even if it is a screw, you try to hit it with the hammer. And eventually, you run out of options. A chiropractor's toolbox looks much different. When traditional medicine has run out of options past medicating, injecting, and surgery, a chiropractor can bring in another box of tools. Traditional doctors often refer to chiropractic care as "not status quo" simply because our tools and methods are not exactly the same. The end goal is always the same….pain free, optimal health for ALL of our patients. The ability to accept and embrace the differences in our paths to reach this goal is so important.

What inspired you to become a Chiropractor?

Dr. Jason Pape*:* I wasn't necessarily one of those people who felt like I had a "calling". Over the course of my life, I was always thinking about becoming some sort of doctor. As a small child, I was interested in pediatrics. As I grew, I took an interest in dentistry and then finally, chiropractic. My parents both saw a chiropractor so I was able to see the benefits firsthand. While I was in school, I was torn between psychology and chiropractic care. I knew I wanted to help people. The theory behind chiropractic really drew me in as I started learning about the integration of our systems and helping them to work together cohesively to create optimal health, and that chiropractic care was about finding the root of the problem. When I began my career, it immediately felt very good to help others in that sort of capacity. Early in my chiropractic journey, I started learning more about holistic medicine and becoming less of just a technician. Many chiropractors don't go beyond the spine or musculoskeletal components. But I realized I had the opportunity to help much more. I got my postgraduate degree in chiropractic sports medicine in 1999 and another in pediatrics over 15 years ago. As I learned more and more, I decided it was my duty to help spread the awareness of the benefits of chiropractic care. There are so many people out there not living life to the fullest due to disease, chronic illness, pain, or even negative thoughts. Everyone deserves the chance to live optimally and I truly believe it is my responsibility to give people this opportunity. It isn't just what I do...it's who I am.

Do you have a specialty when it comes to chiropractic care or functional medicine?

Dr. Jason Pape: One of the things that I am very passionate about, especially over the last few years, is the ketogenic diet and ketones. This comes into play a lot with my patients who are interested in weight loss or just from a functional medicine perspective in general. By nature, we are hunter/gatherers. This is our genetic makeup and it has not changed even though our lifestyles are different now. A hunter/gatherer spends 70% of the time using ketones for fuel, not glucose. But because we don't starve and we eat carbs now, we almost never see ketones anymore. We live in glucose based metabolisms. This is not how it was meant to be. Our bodies function best with the proper fuel source of ketones. The only way to get into this state nowadays is either through a ketogenic lifestyle (which is a high fat, low carb, moderate protein diet) fasting or drinking them in the form of pure therapeutic ketones. I promote a very clean Keto diet. I have even trademarked a name for myself "Dr. Ketone", because of what a huge piece this is when it comes to health and wellness. Again, if we bring the body back to what it is supposed to be doing, things naturally improve. I provide my patients with the latest research on ketones and the ketogenic lifestyle, how to do it the right way, and the numerous health benefits associated with it.

What's the most important thing people should consider when choosing a Chiropractor?

Dr. Jason Pape: Over the years, I have found the best way to find a chiropractor is through a referral. If someone can refer you who truly loves their chiropractor and may even have a similar kind of issue to the one you are experiencing, this is a great way to find one. Obviously, you can search online, but you may not get the whole picture. A solid referral from someone you trust is usually your best option. My practice has grown exponentially through referrals.

If you are searching on your own, do your research. What do their profiles look like and what are they out there doing? For example, I am very visible on Facebook and other social media platforms. I do a lot of Facebook lives and do my best to educate the public via these avenues. Potential patients can easily see what I am all about and make an educated decision about allowing me to guide them on their journey to optimal health.

How can someone find out more about you, your practice, how you can help, and how to reach you?

Dr. Jason Pape*:* People typically reach me via a call to the office or through my website. My staff is highly trained to guide patients through that first call and talk about the problems they are experiencing and ways we can help. Sometimes patients with several issues are confused as to where to begin and a short consultation with me in person or on the phone is always an option as well. We want each patient to feel confident about getting started in the office and have a framework for what to expect.

JASON I. PAPE, D.C., C.C.S.P., C.A.C.C.P.

Owner/Chiropractor

The Vitality Center and Thrive Chiropractic and Wellness

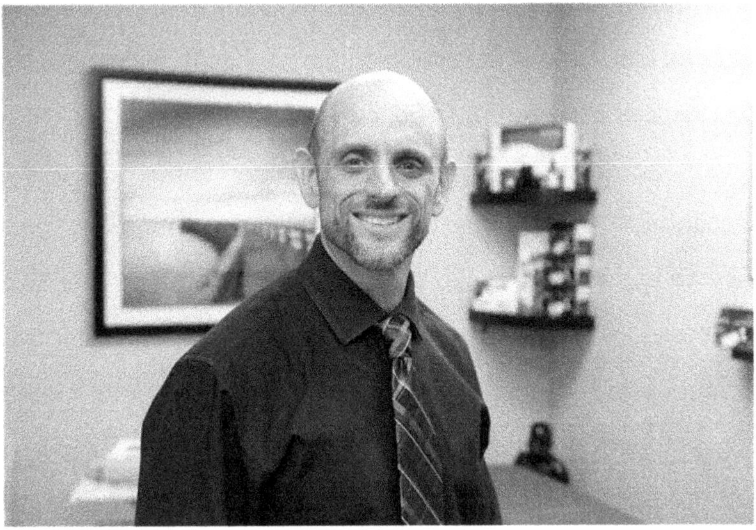

Dr. Jason I. Pape is a chiropractor and functional medicine doctor and graduated Summa Cum Laude from New York Chiropractic College in 1998. Dr. Pape believes strongly in the body's ability to, when given the proper nutrition, neurological input and biomechanical stability, not only heal itself, but to exist in a state of optimal function. Believing in educating not just his patients, but also those outside of his clinic's walls, Dr. Pape hopes to help shape a new paradigm of health. Understanding that the human body works as a complex interplay of intricate and intimately related systems, he focuses his patient care and community education on these principles. Knowing that working to balance these systems with proper diet, nutrition, supplementation, neurological input, chiropractic care and positive mindset, Dr. Pape understands that you can achieve true optimization of health and wellbeing. As much as he believes in educating others on the benefits of holistic health care, Dr. Pape is constantly continuing his own education, understanding that he needs to continue to expand his own knowledge base to best help patients to achieve optimal wellness. While holding post-graduate degrees in both pediatrics and sports medicine as well as various certifications in chiropractic and soft tissue techniques, he also is an expert in neurosensory integration, neurofeedback, methylation, and the paleo and ketogenic diets, and is currently finishing two more post-graduate degrees in functional medicine. Dr. Pape believes that it is his duty to help others to strive to become the best versions of themselves.

WEBSITE: vitalitycenterli.com; drketone.com

EMAIL: wellspine@gmail.com

FACEBOOK: https://www.facebook.com/TrueWellness;

https://www.facebook.com/VitalityCenterLI

OFFICE: 631-864-2784

INSTAGRAM: @thevitalitycenter; @drketone; @jipape

Conversation with Dr. Keta Patel

Tell us about your practice and the type of patients you serve.

Dr. Keta Patel: I am the owner and founder of Excel Wellness Center. As well as being a chiropractic physician, I also practice functional medicine. My clients are people who are looking for a natural way of gaining the best health possible. They may have tried many different avenues and traditional medicines, but are still unable to find that root cause and feel "alive". I have many patients who simply want to be free from medication and I can help with that as well.

What is functional medicine and how does it relate to chiropractic care?

Dr. Keta Patel*:* Chiropractors are considered "holistic practitioners". We believe in leading a healthy lifestyle and eating right in order to achieve the best overall health possible. Functional wellness incorporates elements such as nutrition, supplements, exercising, and working on stress levels so that patients can feel empowered by having a grasp on their own health. By doing these things well, people can eliminate the need for medication. We coach each patient along their journey in order to help them achieve goals. Though functional medicine is not a "quick fix" like medication, it is well worth the time and effort. Patients can gain years in their life where they feel like they are *actually* living. They won't just be sitting and watching their grandchildren play. They will feel good enough to engage and get right down on the floor to play with them. I always say that chiropractic helps me take care of my patient's external needs like aches and pains, while functional medicine takes care of the inside. It is an ideal, holistic approach to health and wellness.

When we talk about functional medicine, the goal is to find the root of the problem. We are not just treating symptoms. For example, if a patient comes in with a thyroid issue that they have been taking medication for, we use state of the art labs to figure out WHY that thyroid may not be functioning well. Perhaps there is an underlying issue in the liver or gut that is impacting the thyroid. Once we find the root cause, everything else falls into place. I tell all of my patients that I won't just treat one issue. Functional medicine allows me to treat the WHOLE person.

What do you feel are the biggest myths out there when it comes to Chiropractic?

Dr. Keta Patel*:* People often say "Once you go to a chiropractor, you HAVE to keep going back all the time." It isn't that you HAVE to, but it is IMPORTANT for you to schedule visits for maintenance purposes. When I adjust or manipulate your back, I am helping the signaling between the brain, spinal cord, and other body parts to function correctly. It is a misconception that chiropractic care only treats aches and pains. Once the aches and pains are gone, it is important to keep all of the systems in our body integrated successfully through maintenance care. In the same way that you would maintain a car on a regular basis to keep it from breaking down, you want to maintain chiropractic care to achieve optimal health.

What inspired you to become a Chiropractor?

Dr. Keta Patel: My inspiration began in high school after seeing my mom go through physical therapy. It really had a big impact on me to see her suffering from pain and then finding relief through therapy and the proper treatments. I was very excited and talked with my brother about going into physical therapy as a career. He suggested chiropractic since I could see my own patients, perform all of the rehab, the therapies, and add on so many other modalities through my education as a doctor. I looked into it and literally fell in love with the concept. Getting people well naturally, holistically, and really teaching them about diet, exercise and all of the fundamental ways to keep our bodies healthy was very exciting for me. I immediately understood the importance of taking it back to the basics, before we became a society that relied on medication. Being able to provide this kind of valuable information to my patients really drove my passion for chiropractic care.

Is there anything else you would like to share?

Dr. Keta Patel: I was invited to speak at Harvard Club of Boston in front of 120+ entrepreneurs. I had the opportunity to speak about my "big why", referring to why I started practicing chiropractic and functional wellness. It was a very inspirational moment for me and I met so many wonderful people. The common denominator between myself and this particular group of people was that we weren't just in business to make money. Each one of us genuinely cares about our clients. I feel this is what sets me apart. I take the time to give each of my patients the care they deserve. I listen, understand, and provide hope that even though they may feel miserable and medicated now, we can work together to make them feel amazing and medication-free.

How can someone find out more about you, your practice, how you can help, and how to reach you?

Dr. Keta Patel: Anyone who wants to find out more about me can go to my website at www.drketa.com, my Facebook page at Excel Wellness Center, or Instagram at excelwellnesscenter. If you wish to speak with me directly, I can be reached by phone at 225-733-1500.

DR. KETA PATEL, DC

Owner/Founder

Excel Wellness Center

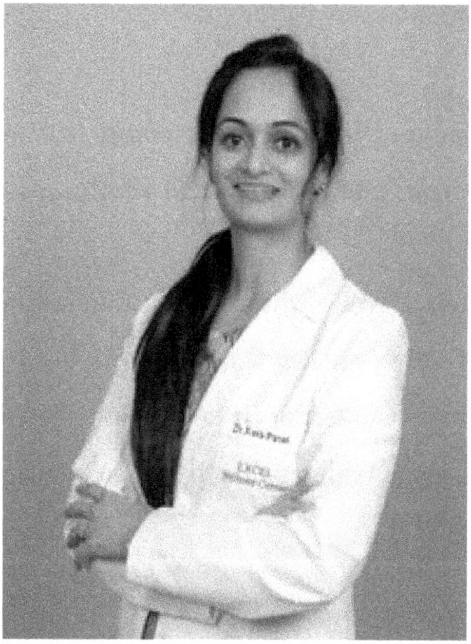

"Hope, a tiny glimpse of light that gives us the strength to persevere in any situation".

Since childhood I have learned, not through words...but by the actions of my biggest mentors...my dad Atul and my mom Renuka... to always work hard, to be passionate and most importantly, to stay hopeful.

So....when it came time to choose a career, I chose to be a chiropractic physician because I was passionate about helping people feel better and seeing that smile on their faces as they walk out of my office pain-free!

About 3 years ago, one of my mentors, my mom got sick....really, really sick!

I saw her transform from being full of life and so active, willing to help anyone and everyone, ready to cook delicious meals for her family...to someone who is scared that she is probably dying, hopeless and weak. She was not able to do things she absolutely enjoyed, like gardening and walking.

I remember the exact moment sitting at my son's swim lessons when I got a call from my dad and he said "Keta, the doctors are saying that your mom may need a lung transplant." I didn't know what to say to him.

I felt so HELPLESS.

"I couldn't help her heal... WHAT??

...but I am a doctor".

You see, when someone gets sick, it's not just their life that changes...their whole family's life changes as well. For a husband, it's the wife. For the children, it's the mother. For grandkids, it's the grandma. For me, it was my best friend, and I was NOT ready to lose her. HOPE!! said that tiny voice inside of me as I searched to find a way to bring my mom BACK. After days of relentless searching and talking to colleagues, I learned about this AMAZING concept of being able to get to the root cause of illness by changing the dysfunction in your body. To be able to transform people's lives, to give them the knowledge to stay healthy and give them a better quality of life...by teaching people the importance of a healthy lifestyle that incorporates a whole person approach and not covering up their symptoms. So it's become my mission to be able to help change not only my mom's health, but to be able to help the lives of people in my community using the knowledge of FUNCTIONAL MEDICINE. It has become my new found passion!

So I stand here today as your Expert Wellness Practitioner because....

HE WHO HAS HEALTH HAS HOPE & HE WHO HAS HOPE HAS EVERYTHING!!

WEBSITE: www.drketa.com

FACEBOOK: Excel Wellness Center

OFFICE: 225-733-1500

INSTAGRAM: @excelwellnesscenter

DR. DEBRA PAVLOVIC

Conversation with Dr. Debra Pavlovic

Tell us about your practice and the type of patients you serve.

Dr. Debra Pavlovic*:* My practice is Atlas Wellness of Lakeland. I've been in Lakeland, FL since 2008. This is actually a second career for me. It all began when I was involved in a tornado at the age of five years old. As a result, I started experiencing chronic migraine headaches. I had them all the way up until the age of 30 when I had my first Atlas correction and they went away. I specifically chose to practice Atlas chiropractic because it is so rare and I wanted to be part of the solution for people with migraine headaches rather than just being a benefactor.

I also specialize in treating anything neurological. I am currently working on my diplomat in the craniocervical junction. I am studying concussions, traumatic brain injuries, and post traumatic stress disorders. I recently witnessed a quadriplegic who is walking and mobile after receiving an Atlas adjustment and working very hard for two years now. He is speaking to others with his condition and giving them hope, revealing that medical doctors don't necessarily have all the answers. It is amazing to see the kind of positive life changes that Atlas adjustments can bring about.

What are some of the most common issues your patients struggle with?

Dr. Debra Pavlovic*:* One of the biggest conditions is an imbalance in the limbic system, which allows information to travel to the brain. Your brain receives nerve signals from joints and muscles that tell the brain where the joints are positioned. When that data gets jumbled up, it starts to change whether the brain is getting correct information. The bottom line is that your head needs to be centered over gravity to maintain balance.

When those tones change, it can cause stressful stimuli for the hypothalamus and the limbic system, which results in a fight or flight response. This increases stress hormones, heart rate, blood pressure, muscle tone, reflex response, adrenaline, and rapid fatigue. It also decreases immune system response, causing you to get sick more often. Digestion and excretion decrease creating issues with the gut. Healing responses decrease. The one that affects my patients the most seems to be the decrease in cognitive function. They complain of feeling "foggy headed" and they simply can't think straight.

One of the things that we're learning is how the gut/ brain connection is really serious. The cranial nerve 10, which is responsible for swallowing, breathing, heart rate, and gut, travels all the way down to the top part of the colon. If you get bad food and toxic waste in your gut, it can literally travel back up to the brainstem through cranial nerve 10. This is causing health issues within the brain for many people. A chiropractor can help get the systems of the body working together in harmony once again.

Can you describe the specific type of chiropractic care that you provide and how it can benefit people?

Dr. Debra Pavlovic*:* Chiropractic wasn't started or designed to cure or treat any illnesses. The cool thing about what I do is putting the bones back where they belong, in order to allow the body to do its job the way it was designed to do it. So when a body is malfunctioning, it's not because the person is lacking a drug. It's not because they're lacking a surgery. It's because the information isn't traveling back and forth properly due to a blockage. The purpose of chiropractic is to locate these misalignments and correct them so the spine is perfectly aligned. Most people don't realize there are about 200 different techniques when it comes to chiropractic care. The upper cervical specific technique is the one that I use. It is called EPIC, which stands for Evolutionary Percussive Instrument Corrections. The amount of force needed is so low that I have adjusted newborns with torticollis and 96 year old ladies with osteoporosis. I am the only chiropractor in my area that uses this technique. It is so gentle that you don't even feel the adjustment, which is wonderful for the very young and very old patients that I serve. Since it is gentle AND effective, I get patients flying in to my Lakeland, FL practice from places all over the globe including Puerto Rico, Italy, and Indiana. They don't mind traveling to get results.

What inspired you to become a chiropractor?

Dr. Debra Pavlovic*:* My husband was diagnosed with MS when we had been married almost three years and I was chaperoning a youth group to Nashville, Tennessee. I met a student from Life University Chiropractic. He told me that there were guys in Jacksonville doing this really strange low force correction at the brainstem and that they were performing a lot of studies with MS patients. Since my husband was recently diagnosed, I thought, well, let's take him there. And the more he talked about it, the more I thought that it could help with my migraine headaches. And just like that, after giving it a try, my migraine headaches, TMJ, and PMS went away. Of thirty MS patients that received this type of chiropractic care, twenty-eight went into remission. My husband and one other did not. The missing ingredient for my husband was diet. I learned this in the last 10 years since he's passed away. I could have helped him to live if I had known then what I know now.. That's kind of sad, but I had to take lemons and turn them into lemonade. I had to make a bad situation turn into something good and worthwhile, by helping others through the power of chiropractic

How can someone find out more about you, your practice, how you can help, and how to reach you?

Dr. Debra Pavlovic*:* You can reach me by text at 863-393-4169 or email at atlasoflakeland@gmail.com.

DR. DEBRA PAVLOVIC, DC

Owner/Chiropractor

Atlas Wellness of Lakeland

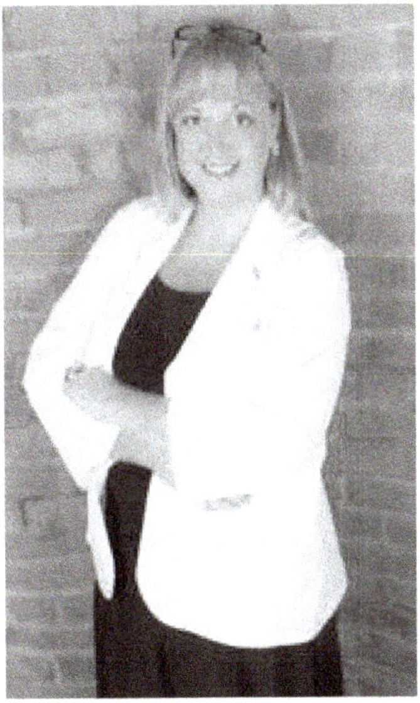

Dr Pavlovic is a very caring and low force chiropractor. She is interested in getting patients well and keeping patients well, without having long care plans. Minerals and nutrition are a big part of her protocol. She is back in Lakeland, Florida following 5 years in South Georgia where she helped her husband finish raising his 3 children. She has returned to the Lakeland community because that is where her heart is. Following the death of her first husband, she chose Lakeland over anywhere in the world. There is no doctor doing what she does in Polk County. If you want to be well or stay well, this is your doctor.

TEXT: 863-393-4169

EMAIL: atlasoflakeland@gmail.com

DR. IAN RAINEY

Conversation with Dr. Ian Rainey

Tell us about your practice and the type of patients you serve.

Dr. Ian Rainey*:* My practice is Rainey Chiropractic and Car Injury Clinic out of Dunedin, Florida, which borders Clearwater. It is a small town close to the beach. I am a second generation chiropractor. My father was a chiropractor and my sister is a chiropractor. I guess you could say it runs in my blood. I have a passion for helping people achieve optimal health. Whether you are trying to get out of pain or simply starting out on a wellness journey to live the best life you can, I can help accomplish these goals through chiropractic care.

Are there any particular specialites you offer at your clinic?

Dr. Ian Rainey: Like I mentioned before, my father is a chiropractor. My mother has owned a health food store for forty years, even before health food was really popular. I have a strong background in nutrition and I will do everything in my power to help people improve their health through diet. A lot of people come into my office with an initial desire to lose weight. Maybe they suffer from knee pain due to the excess weight, and helping them to lose a few pounds really reduces that inflammation in the body and helps them to see how much better they can feel. Weight loss is just a great entry point because I generally help my patients lose twenty to forty pounds in just 4 weeks. Helping people safely lose this weight in just one month is a wonderful start to really transforming the quality of their lives.

What are the most common issues that patients are struggling with when they come to see you?

Dr. Ian Rainey*:* Most typically I am treating neck and back pain. Those are the two main conditions that chiropractors are known for being excellent at treating and helping people to resolve. I also help with a lot of sciatica, which is radiating pain through the fingers, toes, or arms. Here in Florida, we see many car accidents, so helping people recover from the after effects of those makes up a majority of my practice as well.

What do you feel are the biggest myths out there when it comes to chiropractic?

Dr. Ian Rainey*:* Many medical doctors think that chiropractors are trying to steal their patients or vice versa. In reality, there is a very small percentage of people who even utilize chiropractic...much smaller than you would think. People simply don't realize that there is a natural way to relieve neck and back pain that does not require drugs or surgery. I make it a priority to work cooperatively with all of the medical doctors in the area because it really provides a great synergy to help people achieve optimal health.

People also worry about chiropractic care being painful. All of the new chiropractic training shows you exactly how to adjust in a very gentle fashion. For people who are concerned about having me adjust their neck, I have a special little tool called the activator. It looks like a spring loaded clicker and it is very fast, yet very gentle. I put it right up to the vertebrae and it applies a quick little force that makes the bone oscillate, or vibrate, if you will. As a result, the muscles start to relax around that bone. You will notice all of a sudden that you get your motion back, the pain goes away, and you just feel a lot better. There are many different approaches I can take to get people feeling better. Especially with the first experience, I take the time to make my patients feel comfortable by explaining everything and discussing a more gentle technique if they have some initial fears.

What inspired you to become a chiropractor?

Dr. Ian Rainey*:* When I was a little kid, I can remember being in my dad's office and it would be completely silent. And I would be sitting there and thinking, "This is so boring. I don't want to do this. I want to be a fireman or a policeman or something really cool." As I got older, I really started to understand and appreciate what my dad was doing. One day, he was in between treating patients at the office and he had a heart attack. That heart attack ended up taking his life. I remember when I went to his funeral, people came up to me and said the most wonderful things about my father. One person said "Your dad saved my life". Another one said "Your dad saved my dog's life." I never even knew that my dad adjusted an animal, but he did and the dog's owner said it was amazing. I started thinking that chiropractic was quite a noble profession. I wanted to be able to touch people's lives and improve their overall health through chiropractic care, just like my father. I decided to go to chiropractic school a little bit later in life and follow in my dad's footsteps.

Is there anything else you would like to share?

Dr. Ian Rainey: Chiropractic is interesting. It is a little bit different from office to office. We all go to school, but there may be 50 different chiropractic techniques that achieve the same objective, which is to remove nerve interference in the body so that the body can express itself at one hundred percent. Though we each may have our own way of doing things, our ultimate goal is always the same...to help people get out of pain, achieve optimal health, or just enjoy life a little more. It's a very unique profession in that you cannot franchise it. One chiropractor may use his hands for adjustments, another may use a tool. One chiropractor may help with weight loss, another may not. It is important that you feel comfortable with the chiropractor you choose to work with and confident in their ability to help with your specific issue. We all want to work with people we can help, and likewise, you should want to go to a practice where you can get the results you expect.

How can someone find out more about you, your practice, how you can help, and how to reach you?

Dr. Ian Rainey*:* My website is raineychiropractic.com. If you would prefer to reach me by phone, the number is 727-314-2663.

DR. IAN RAINEY, DC

Owner/Chiropractor

Rainey Chiropractic and Car Injury Clinic

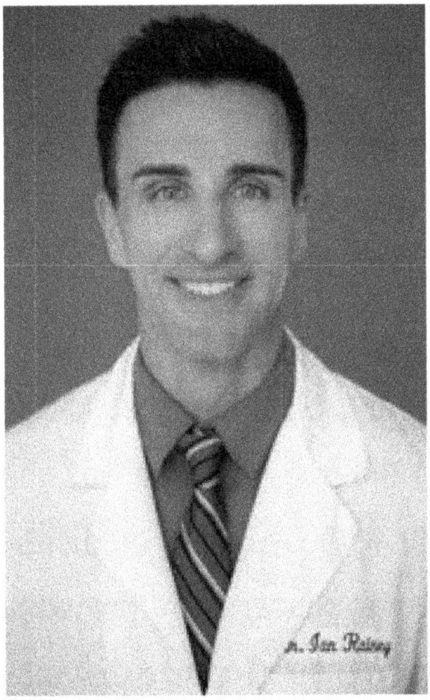

Dr. Ian Rainey, D.C. graduated from Miami University and received his doctorate from Life University in Atlanta, Ga. He has received extensive post-doctorate education and training in Functional Medicine and Nutrition through various seminars, workshops and university training. Dr. Rainey is a licensed doctor of chiropractic in the states of Ohio and Florida. He sits on the board for Spinal Missions. Spinal Missions is a non-profit organization of chiropractic doctors, students and others that have a burning desire to aid people of underprivileged nations in addressing health care issues.

Dr. Rainey is an expert and international lecturer on functional blood chemistry analysis. He specializes in identifying the underlying factors in chronic disease and customizing health programs for these conditions such as thyroid issues, autoimmune, hormonal dysfunctions, digestive disorders, diabetes, heart disease and fibromyalgia. He is among the doctors of the future.

We utilize a unique approach that seeks to discover and correct dysfunction within the body. Instead of chasing symptoms or masking symptoms with drugs or medications, we get to the core of your particular concerns by providing the body what it is lacking and removing interference that may be preventing the body from expressing optimal health.

WEBSITE: raineychiropractic.com

OFFICE: 727-314-2663

ABOUT THE PUBLISHER

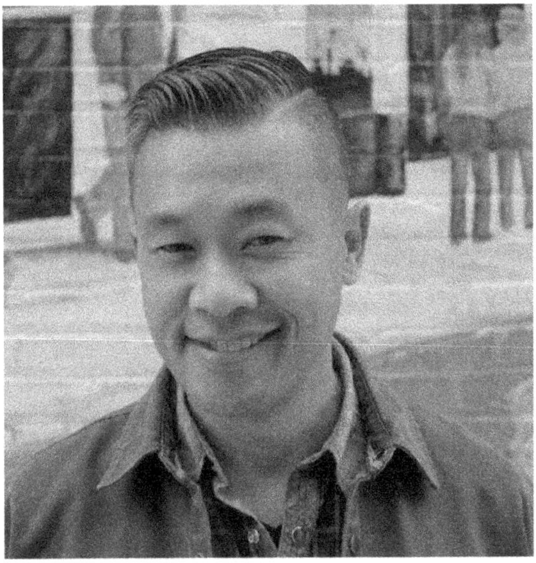

Mark Imperial is a Best-Selling Author, Syndicated Business Columnist, Syndicated Radio Host, and internationally recognized Stage, Screen, and Radio Host of numerous business shows spotlighting leading experts, entrepreneurs, and business celebrities.

His passion is discovering noteworthy business owners, professionals, experts, and leaders who do great work, and sharing their stories and secrets to their success with the world on his syndicated radio program titled "Remarkable Radio".

Mark is also the media marketing strategist and voice for some of the world's most famous brands. You can hear his voice over the airwaves weekly on Chicago radio and worldwide on iHeart Radio.

Mark is a Karate black belt, teaches kickboxing, loves Thai food, House Music, and his favorite TV shows are infomercials.

Learn more:
www.MarkImperial.com
www.ImperialAction.com
www.RemarkableRadioShow.com

www.ingramcontent.com/pod-product-compliance
Lightning Source LLC
Chambersburg PA
CBHW071139280326
41935CB00010B/1293
* 9 7 8 1 7 3 2 3 7 6 3 5 9 *